CHRONIC PAIN

A Guide to Alternative and Complementary Therapies

Susan Robbie

To my children, you do yourselves incredibly proud.

Pain is like fire; it burns everything it touches, but some things emerge from the fire more beautiful than they were before.

PAULO COELHO

CONTENTS

PREFACE

The patient's experience, often overlooked, is as crucial, if not more so, than the diagnosis, treatment, and cure. This guide stems from a conversation with a former nurse, who lamented the inadequate attention given to chronic pain management, particularly, the role magnesium can play. I hope it brings even a single patient some relief, for then it will have served its purpose.

CHAPTER 1: UNDERSTANDING CHRONIC PAIN

"Pain is inevitable. Suffering is optional." - Haruki Murakami

What Is Chronic Pain?

Chronic pain is a major health problem that affects millions of people around the world, and many people are looking for holistic, alternative and complementary therapies to help manage their pain.

It is a complex and multifaceted condition, defined as pain that persists for longer than three months, and it can have a profound impact on a person's physical, emotional, and social well-being.

The Different Types Of Chronic Pain

There are many different causes of chronic pain, including arthritis, back pain, and fibromyalgia. Chronic pain can also be caused by nerve damage, cancer, and other medical conditions.

The symptoms of chronic pain can vary depending on the underlying cause. However, some common symptoms include, pain that:

- lasts for longer than three months
- is localised to a specific area or widespread throughout the body
- is constant or intermittent
- is described as aching, burning, shooting, or tingling
- is accompanied by other symptoms, such as fatigue, sleep disturbances, and mood changes

The Impact Of Chronic Pain On Quality Of Life

Chronic pain can have a significant impact on a person's life. It can make it difficult to work, sleep, and enjoy activities that you once enjoyed. Chronic pain can also lead to depression, anxiety, and social isolation.

There is no single cure for chronic pain, but there are a variety of treatments that can help manage symptoms. Treatment approaches often involve a combination of therapies, including:

- Medication: Pain medications, such as nonsteroidal anti-inflammatory drugs (NSAIDs), opioids, and antidepressants, may be prescribed to manage pain symptoms.
- Physical therapy: Physical therapy can help improve muscle

strength, flexibility, and range of motion, which can help reduce pain and improve function.

- Cognitive-behavioural therapy (CBT): CBT can help individuals develop coping mechanisms for managing pain and improving emotional well-being.
- Complementary and alternative therapies: Some complementary and alternative or non-pharmacological therapies, such as acupuncture, massage therapy, and yoga, may provide additional pain relief and symptom management.

Living with chronic pain requires ongoing management and adaptation. Individuals with chronic pain may need to make lifestyle changes to accommodate their pain, such as adjusting their work schedule, limiting physical activities, and adopting relaxation techniques. Support groups and pain management programs can also provide valuable resources and guidance for coping with chronic pain.

With proper management and support, individuals with chronic pain can learn to live fulfilling and meaningful lives.

The Importance Of Self-Management

Self-managing chronic pain is crucial for several reasons:

1. Empowerment and Control: Self-management allows individuals to take charge of their pain, rather than feeling helpless or reliant solely on healthcare providers. This sense of empowerment can boost confidence and self-efficacy, leading to better pain management outcomes.
2. Tailored Approach: Chronic pain is highly individual, so self-management enables individuals to personalise their strategies based on their unique experiences and needs. This personalised approach often leads to more effective pain

relief and symptom management.

3. Proactive Prevention: Self-management encourages individuals to be proactive in identifying and addressing pain triggers and early warning signs. This proactive approach helps prevent pain flare-ups and reduces the overall burden of chronic pain.

4. Improved Quality of Life: By effectively managing pain, individuals can experience a significant improvement in their quality of life. Self-management allows them to participate in activities they enjoy, maintain work and relationships, and live a more fulfilling life.

5. Reduced Healthcare Costs: Self-management can reduce the need for frequent healthcare visits and expensive treatments, leading to lower healthcare costs. This is particularly important for individuals with chronic pain who may face financial strain due to their condition.

6. Holistic Well-being: Self-management often involves incorporating lifestyle changes and complementary therapies, promoting overall well-being beyond pain relief. This holistic approach addresses the physical, emotional, and psychological aspects of chronic pain, leading to a more balanced and healthy lifestyle.

In summary, self-management of chronic pain is essential for empowering individuals, tailoring pain management strategies, preventing pain flare-ups, improving quality of life, reducing healthcare costs, and promoting holistic well-being. By taking an active role in managing their pain, individuals can achieve a greater sense of control and live a more fulfilling life.

According to a 2020 survey by the American Chronic Pain Association, 74% of people with chronic pain reported using alternative therapies to manage their pain. The most common alternative therapies used were exercise (59%), diet (53%), and yoga (34%) (Chronic Pain Facts and Figures Survey. Retrieved from https://www.acpanow.com/).

CHAPTER 2: EXERCISE AS AN ALTERNATIVE THERAPY

"The pain you feel today is the strength you feel tomorrow." - Robert Tew

The Benefits Of Exercise For Chronic Pain

Exercise can be a helpful tool for managing chronic pain. It can help to reduce pain symptoms, improve flexibility and range of motion, and boost your mood. Exercise can also help to prevent muscle atrophy and osteoporosis, which are common complications of chronic pain.

Here are some of the benefits of exercise for chronic pain:

- Reduces pain: Exercise releases endorphins, which have natural pain-relieving properties. It can also help to reduce inflammation, which is a major contributor to chronic pain.
- Improves flexibility and range of motion: Exercise helps to keep your muscles and joints limber, which can help to reduce pain and improve your ability to move around.
- Boosts mood: Exercise releases endorphins, which have

mood-boosting effects. It can also help to reduce stress and anxiety, which are often associated with chronic pain.

- Prevents muscle atrophy and osteoporosis: Muscle atrophy is the loss of muscle mass, which can occur as a result of chronic pain. Osteoporosis is a condition that weakens bones, making them more susceptible to fracture. Exercise can help to prevent both of these conditions.
- Improves sleep: Exercise can help to improve sleep quality, which is often disrupted by chronic pain.
- Reduces fatigue: Exercise can help to reduce fatigue, which is a common symptom of chronic pain.
- Improves overall health: Exercise has a number of other health benefits, including reducing the risk of heart disease, stroke, and type 2 diabetes.

Types Of Exercise For Chronic Pain

Here are some types of exercise that are beneficial for chronic pain:

- Low-impact aerobic exercise: This type of exercise is easy on your joints and can be done for extended periods. Examples include walking, swimming, and biking.
- Strength training: This type of exercise helps to build muscle strength, which can help to support your joints and reduce pain. Examples include lifting weights, using resistance bands, and bodyweight exercises.
- Flexibility exercises: This type of exercise helps to improve your range of motion and can make it easier to move around. Examples include yoga, tai chi, and Pilates.
- Balance exercises: This type of exercise helps to improve your balance and coordination, which can help to prevent falls. Examples include standing on one leg, walking heel-to-toe, and using a balance ball.

- Water exercises: Water exercises are gentle on your joints and can provide support while you exercise. Examples include water aerobics, swimming laps, and aqua jogging.

How To Start An Exercise Program For Chronic Pain

If you are living with chronic pain, talk to your doctor about starting an exercise program. They can help you to develop a safe and effective program that is right for you.

Here are some tips for starting an exercise program for chronic pain:

- Start slowly: Don't try to do too much too soon. Start with a few minutes of exercise each day and gradually increase the amount of time you exercise as you get stronger.
- Choose activities that you enjoy: If you enjoy the activities you do, you are more likely to stick with them. There are many different types of exercise, so find something that you enjoy and that fits into your lifestyle.
- Listen to your body: Pay attention to how your body feels during and after exercise. If you experience pain, stop the activity and rest.
- Work with a qualified professional: A physical therapist or personal trainer can help you to develop a safe and effective exercise program that is right for you.

With a little effort, exercise can be a helpful tool for managing chronic pain and improving your quality of life.

Safety Tips For Exercising With Chronic Pain

It's important to take precautions to avoid aggravating your pain or causing further injury. Here are some safety tips for exercising with chronic pain:

1. Talk to your doctor: Before starting any new exercise program, consult with your doctor to discuss your specific condition and limitations. They can provide guidance on safe and appropriate exercises for you.
2. Start slowly and gradually increase intensity: Begin with low-impact exercises for short durations and gradually increase the intensity and duration as your tolerance improves. Don't push yourself too hard too soon.
3. Choose low-impact exercises: Opt for low-impact exercises that put minimal stress on your joints, such as walking, swimming, cycling, or water aerobics. Avoid high-impact activities like running or jumping until your pain is under better control.
4. Warm up and cool down: Always warm up before exercising to prepare your muscles and joints, and cool down afterward to promote recovery and prevent stiffness.
5. Listen to your body: Pay attention to any pain signals during or after exercise. If you experience pain, stop the activity and rest. Don't disregard pain as a sign of weakness or a hurdle to overcome.
6. Wear supportive footwear: Proper footwear can make a significant difference in reducing pain and preventing injuries. Choose shoes that provide good support, cushioning, and fit your feet well.
7. Modify exercises as needed: Adapt exercises to suit your pain levels and limitations. For instance, instead of doing deep lunges, try shallow lunges or stationary lunges with support.
8. Use proper form and technique: Maintain proper form and technique during exercises to avoid strain and injury. If you're unsure about proper form, consider seeking guidance from a physical therapist or personal trainer.

9. Take breaks when needed: Don't hesitate to take breaks during exercise if you feel pain or fatigue. Breaks allow your body to rest and recover, preventing further discomfort.
10. Maintain a healthy lifestyle: Combine exercise with a healthy diet and adequate sleep to promote overall well-being and support your body's recovery process.

Remember, exercise should be enjoyable and not a source of additional pain. If you experience persistent pain or discomfort, consult your doctor or a physical therapist for personalised guidance and adjustments to your exercise program.

CHAPTER 3: DIET AS AN ALTERNATIVE THERAPY

"Pain is a signal that something is wrong, a message that something needs to change. It is not something to be avoided or ignored, but rather something to be listened to and understood."
- Rachel Naomi Remen

The Role Of Diet In Chronic Pain Management

Diet plays a crucial role in chronic pain management, influencing both the intensity of pain and overall well-being. A well-balanced and nutrient-rich diet can help reduce inflammation, improve mood, and support the body's natural healing processes. There are foods to eat and those to avoid, for helping to manage chronic pain.

Reducing Inflammation:

Chronic pain is often linked to inflammation, which contributes to pain signals and tissue damage. A diet rich in anti-inflammatory foods can help reduce inflammation and alleviate pain symptoms. These foods include:

- Fruits and vegetables: Fruits and vegetables are packed with antioxidants and phytonutrients that have anti-inflammatory properties. Aim for a variety of colourful fruits and vegetables, such as berries, leafy greens, tomatoes, and bell peppers.
- Fatty fish: Fatty fish like salmon, tuna, and mackerel contain omega-3 fatty acids, which have potent anti-inflammatory effects. Aim to consume at least two servings of fatty fish per week.
- Whole grains: Whole grains, including brown rice, quinoa, and oats, provide fibre and nutrients that support anti-inflammatory processes. Choose whole grains over refined grains whenever possible.
- Herbs and spices: Certain herbs and spices, such as turmeric, ginger, and garlic, have anti-inflammatory properties. Incorporate these spices into your cooking for added flavour and health benefits.

"Inflammation is the foundation of all chronic disease. If we can reduce inflammation, we can prevent and reverse chronic disease." - Tim Noakes

Tim Noakes believes that a low-carbohydrate, high-fat diet could help to reduce inflammation and improve overall health, this is due to the importance he places on the role of inflammation in the development of chronic diseases like heart disease, diabetes, and cancer. Have a look at his book, The Real Meal Revolution: The Noakes Foundation Guide to Low-Carb, High-Fat Eating. Myburgh Publishing (2013).

Improving Mood and Overall Well-being:

Chronic pain can significantly impact mood and overall well-being. A healthy diet can help regulate mood, improve sleep, and boost energy levels, which can contribute to pain management and overall quality of life.

- Balanced meals: Aim for balanced meals that include protein, carbohydrates, and healthy fats to provide sustained energy and prevent blood sugar swings that can affect mood.
- Regular hydration: Drink plenty of water throughout the day to stay hydrated and support body functions. Dehydration can contribute to fatigue and worsen pain perception.
- Adequate sleep: Adequate sleep is essential for pain management and overall well-being. Aim for 7-8 hours of quality sleep each night to promote healing and reduce pain sensitivity.
- Stress management: Chronic stress can exacerbate pain symptoms. Incorporate stress-management techniques, such as yoga, meditation, or deep breathing exercises, into your daily routine.

Dietary Considerations for Specific Pain Conditions:

Certain dietary modifications may be beneficial for individuals with specific chronic pain conditions. For instance:

- Arthritis: A diet rich in omega-3 fatty acids, vitamin D, and calcium may help reduce joint inflammation and pain associated with arthritis.
- Chronic back pain: A diet that includes plenty of fruits, vegetables, and whole grains can help reduce inflammation and support muscle function, which may contribute to pain relief for chronic back pain. Additionally, a diet rich in omega-3 fatty acids may help reduce inflammation and pain associated with chronic back pain.
- Chronic fatigue syndrome (CFS): A diet that includes plenty of fruits, vegetables, and whole grains, and limits processed foods, sugary drinks, and caffeine, may help improve energy levels and reduce fatigue associated with CFS.

- Endometriosis: A diet that includes plenty of fruits, vegetables, and whole grains, and limits processed foods, red meat, and dairy, may help reduce inflammation and pain associated with endometriosis.
- Fibromyalgia: A diet low in gluten, processed foods, and artificial sweeteners may help reduce symptoms such as muscle pain, fatigue, and digestive issues associated with fibromyalgia.
- Irritable bowel syndrome (IBS): A low-FODMAP diet, which eliminates certain types of carbohydrates that can trigger IBS symptoms, may help reduce bloating, diarrhoea, and abdominal pain associated with IBS.
- Migraines: A diet that avoids trigger foods, such as cheese, chocolate, and alcohol, may help reduce the frequency and severity of migraines. Additionally, a diet rich in magnesium and riboflavin may help prevent migraine attacks.
- Neuropathic pain: A diet rich in B vitamins, particularly B12, may help support nerve function and reduce pain associated with neuropathic conditions.

It is important to note that these are just general recommendations, and individual needs may vary. Remember, dietary changes should be implemented gradually and under the guidance of a healthcare professional or registered dietitian. They can help you create a personalised plan that addresses your specific pain condition and overall health needs.

Dietary Supplements For Chronic Pain

Several dietary supplements are available for chronic pain management. These supplements may help reduce pain, improve function, and enhance overall well-being. However, it is crucial to consult with a healthcare professional before taking any supplements, as they may interact with medications or have potential side effects.

Commonly Used Supplements for Chronic Pain:

1. Omega-3 fatty acids: Omega-3 fatty acids, particularly EPA and DHA found in fish oil, have anti-inflammatory properties that may help reduce pain and improve function in individuals with chronic pain conditions like arthritis and fibromyalgia.
2. Glucosamine and chondroitin: These supplements are commonly used for osteoarthritis, the most prevalent form of arthritis. They are believed to provide joint lubrication and reduce pain.
3. Turmeric: Turmeric contains curcumin, a compound with potent anti-inflammatory and antioxidant properties. Studies suggest that curcumin may help reduce pain and improve function in individuals with arthritis and other chronic pain conditions.
4. SAM-e (S-adenosylmethionine): SAM-e is a naturally occurring molecule involved in various bodily processes, including pain regulation. Studies suggest that SAM-e may help reduce pain and improve mood in individuals with osteoarthritis and fibromyalgia.
5. B vitamins: B vitamins, particularly B6, B12, and folic acid, are essential for nerve function. Deficiencies in these vitamins may contribute to neuropathic pain. Supplementation may help improve nerve function and reduce pain in individuals with neuropathic conditions.
6. Magnesium: Magnesium is a mineral involved in muscle and nerve function. Studies suggest that magnesium supplementation may help reduce muscle pain and improve sleep in individuals with fibromyalgia. See further information, below.
7. Vitamin D: Vitamin D plays a role in bone health and inflammation. Studies suggest that vitamin D supplementation may help reduce pain and improve function in individuals with arthritis and fibromyalgia.

8.   Probiotics: Probiotics are live bacteria that support gut health. Studies suggest that probiotics may help reduce inflammation and pain in individuals with inflammatory bowel disease and fibromyalgia.

9. Coenzyme Q10 (CoQ10): CoQ10 is an antioxidant that plays a role in energy production. Studies suggest that CoQ10 supplementation may help reduce pain and improve function in individuals with fibromyalgia.

Important Considerations:

- Supplement Quality: Choose high-quality supplements from reputable brands to ensure purity and potency.
- Individual Variability: Effectiveness of supplements may vary depending on the underlying pain condition and individual response.
- Potential Interactions: Consult with a healthcare professional to assess potential interactions with medications or other supplements.
- Healthcare Guidance: Always seek guidance from a healthcare professional before starting any new supplements, especially if you have any underlying health conditions or are taking medications.

Remember, dietary supplements should not replace conventional pain management strategies, such as exercise, physical therapy, and medication when prescribed by a healthcare professional.

A Spotlight on Magnesium:

Magnesium is a crucial mineral that plays a vital role in various bodily functions, including muscle and nerve function, blood sugar control, and blood pressure regulation. Studies suggest that magnesium may also have beneficial effects in managing chronic pain.

Mechanisms of Magnesium's Pain-Relieving Effects

Magnesium is believed to exert its pain-relieving effects through several mechanisms:

1. Blocking NMDA Receptors: Magnesium acts as a voltage-gated antagonist of N-methyl-D-aspartate (NMDA) receptors, which are involved in pain transmission. By blocking NMDA receptors, magnesium can reduce the influx of calcium ions into nerve cells, thereby dampening pain signals.
2. Reducing Central Sensitisation: Central sensitisation occurs when the nervous system becomes hypersensitive to pain signals, leading to increased pain intensity and duration. Magnesium is thought to reduce central sensitisation by modulating the activity of NMDA receptors and other signalling molecules involved in pain pathways.
3. Anti-inflammatory Effects: Magnesium possesses anti-inflammatory properties that can contribute to pain relief. Inflammation is a common component of chronic pain conditions, and magnesium can help reduce inflammation by modulating the activity of inflammatory cells and signalling molecules.
4. Muscle Relaxation: Magnesium plays a role in muscle relaxation, and its deficiency can contribute to muscle tension and pain. Supplementation with magnesium can help relax muscles and reduce muscle-related pain.

Evidence Supporting Magnesium for Chronic Pain Management

Several studies have investigated the effects of magnesium supplementation on chronic pain management. While research is ongoing, some promising findings suggest that magnesium may provide pain relief for various chronic pain conditions:

1. Fibromyalgia: Studies have shown that magnesium supplementation can improve pain symptoms, fatigue, and sleep quality in individuals with fibromyalgia.
2. Neuropathic Pain: Magnesium has demonstrated pain-

relieving effects in neuropathic pain, a type of pain caused by nerve damage.

3. Migraines: Magnesium supplementation may help reduce migraine frequency and severity.
4. Menstrual Cramps: Magnesium may help alleviate menstrual cramps and associated pain.
5. Chronic Back Pain: Magnesium supplementation may provide pain relief and improve function in individuals with chronic back pain.

Recommended Magnesium Dosage for Chronic Pain

The recommended daily intake of magnesium for adults is 400-420 milligrams for men and 310-320 milligrams for women. However, higher doses may be needed for individuals with chronic pain. It is important to consult with a healthcare professional to determine the appropriate magnesium dosage for your specific needs.

Overall, magnesium is a promising natural treatment for chronic pain management. Its ability to block NMDA receptors, reduce central sensitisation, and exert anti-inflammatory effects makes it a potentially valuable tool for alleviating pain symptoms and improving overall quality of life in individuals with chronic pain conditions.

Tips For Creating A Healthy Diet For Chronic Pain

Some additional tips for creating a healthy diet for chronic pain management:

1. Identify food triggers: Keep a food diary to identify foods that may worsen your pain. Avoiding these triggers can help reduce pain flares and improve overall well-being.

2. Practise mindful eating: Pay attention to hunger cues and eat slowly to savour your food and prevent overeating. Mindful eating can help regulate blood sugar levels, improve digestion, and reduce stress, all of which contribute to pain management.

3. Cook more meals at home: Cooking at home gives you control over ingredients and portion sizes, allowing you to create healthier meals that align with your pain management goals.

4. Plan your meals: Planning your meals ahead of time can help you make healthier choices and avoid impulsive decisions that might exacerbate pain.

5. Make gradual changes: Don't try to overhaul your entire diet overnight. Make small, gradual changes that you can maintain over time.

6. Seek support: Consult with a registered dietitian or nutritionist for personalised guidance on creating a healthy diet tailored to your specific pain condition and overall health needs.

7. Combine diet with other healthy habits: Combine a healthy diet with regular exercise, adequate sleep, stress management techniques, and proper pain management strategies for a comprehensive approach to chronic pain management.

Remember, consistency is key when implementing dietary changes for chronic pain management. Small, sustainable changes over time can have a significant impact on your pain levels, overall health, and quality of life.

CHAPTER 4: YOGA AND MINDFULNESS AS ALTERNATIVE THERAPIES

"Pain is not a punishment; it is a teacher. It is here to teach us something about ourselves, about life, and about the world around us." - Eckhart Tolle

The Benefits Of Yoga And Mindfulness For Chronic Pain

Yoga and mindfulness practices offer a range of benefits for individuals living with chronic pain, providing both physical and mental relief. These practices can help reduce pain symptoms, improve flexibility, enhance mood, and promote overall well-being.

Physical Benefits:

1. Reduced Pain Perception: Yoga and mindfulness can help modulate the brain's pain response, reducing the intensity

of perceived pain. Gentle stretching and movement in yoga poses can improve circulation, release endorphins, and promote muscle relaxation, all of which contribute to pain reduction.

2. Improved Flexibility and Range of Motion: Yoga poses focus on stretching and strengthening muscles, leading to increased flexibility and range of motion in joints. This can help reduce stiffness, improve posture, and make everyday activities easier, reducing pain associated with limited movement.

3. Enhanced Physical Function: Regular yoga practice can strengthen muscles, improve balance, and coordination, enhancing overall physical function. This can reduce reliance on pain medication and improve the ability to perform daily activities without discomfort.

Mental and Emotional Benefits:

1. Reduced Stress and Anxiety: Chronic pain often coexists with stress and anxiety, which can exacerbate pain symptoms. Mindfulness techniques like meditation and breathwork can help reduce stress hormones, promote relaxation, and manage anxiety, leading to a calmer and more pain-tolerant state of mind.

2. Improved Mood and Emotional Well-being: Yoga and mindfulness can promote positive emotions, reduce feelings of helplessness and depression, and enhance overall emotional well-being. This can help individuals cope with chronic pain more effectively and maintain a positive outlook.

3. Increased Self-awareness and Body Acceptance: Mindfulness practices encourage present-moment awareness, helping individuals become more attuned to their bodies and pain sensations. This can lead to better understanding of pain triggers, improved body acceptance, and a greater sense of self-control in managing pain.

Integration into Chronic Pain Management:

Yoga and mindfulness can be effectively integrated into a comprehensive chronic pain management plan alongside other modalities like medication, physical therapy, and cognitive behavioural therapy. These practices can complement traditional treatments by providing holistic relief that addresses both physical and mental aspects of chronic pain.

Here are some additional tips for incorporating yoga and mindfulness into chronic pain management:

1. Start slowly and gradually: Begin with gentle yoga poses and mindfulness techniques that suit your pain level and physical limitations.
2. Seek guidance from a qualified instructor: Find a yoga instructor experienced in teaching individuals with chronic pain to ensure proper alignment and modifications.
3. Practice regularly: Consistency is key to reaping the benefits of yoga and mindfulness. Aim for regular practice, even if it's just for a few minutes each day.
4. Listen to your body: Pay attention to your body's signals and adjust poses or breathing exercises as needed to avoid pain or discomfort.
5. Combine with other modalities: Integrate yoga and mindfulness into your existing chronic pain management plan, working with your healthcare provider to determine the most effective approach for you.

Yoga and mindfulness offer a non-pharmacological and complementary approach to chronic pain management, providing both physical and mental relief. By incorporating these practices into your routine, you can enhance your overall well-being, improve your ability to cope with pain, and lead a more fulfilling life.

Types Of Yoga For Chronic Pain

There are numerous yoga styles, each with its own focus and benefits. Here's a description of some types of yoga that are effective for managing chronic pain:

1. Hatha Yoga: Hatha yoga is a foundational style that emphasises physical postures (asanas) and breathing exercises (pranayama). Hatha yoga's emphasis on stretching and strengthening muscles can help reduce pain and improve flexibility, while the breathing exercises can help promote relaxation and reduce stress, both of which contribute to pain management.
2. Yin Yoga: Yin yoga focuses on holding poses for longer durations, typically 3-5 minutes, to target deep connective tissues, ligaments, and fascia. This slow, deep stretching can help improve flexibility, reduce stiffness, and promote relaxation, making it beneficial for chronic pain conditions like arthritis and fibromyalgia.
3. Restorative Yoga: Restorative yoga utilises props such as bolsters, blankets, and blocks to support the body in comfortable, passive poses. This gentle and supported practice promotes deep relaxation, reduces stress, and encourages a sense of calmness, which can be helpful for individuals dealing with chronic pain and its associated stress and anxiety.
4. Iyengar Yoga: Iyengar yoga is known for its emphasis on precise alignment and the use of props to support the body in poses. This precision and support can help individuals with chronic pain modify poses to suit their limitations and avoid pain while still reaping the benefits of yoga.
5. Viniyoga Yoga: Viniyoga yoga is a therapeutic approach that emphasises breath-synchronised movement. This mindful practice encourages individuals to move at their own pace,

aligning movement with breath, which can help reduce strain and discomfort while promoting flexibility, strength, and body awareness.

It is important to choose a yoga style that suits your individual needs and preferences. If you have chronic pain, it is advisable to consult with a healthcare professional before starting any new exercise program, including yoga. They can help you determine the most appropriate style and provide guidance on modifications to suit your limitations.

Mindfulness Techniques For Chronic Pain

Mindfulness techniques can be a valuable tool for managing chronic pain, offering a non-pharmacological approach to reducing pain intensity, improving mood, and enhancing overall well-being. These techniques focus on cultivating present-moment awareness and acceptance, helping individuals become more attuned to their bodies and thoughts without judgement.

Here are some effective mindfulness techniques for chronic pain:

1. Body Scan Meditation: Body scan meditation involves systematically focusing attention on different parts of the body, noticing sensations without judgement. This practice can help individuals become more aware of their pain sensations, allowing them to observe and accept them without feeling overwhelmed.
2. Mindful Breathing: Mindful breathing exercises, such as diaphragmatic breathing, can help reduce stress, promote relaxation, and improve pain perception. By focusing on the natural rhythm of breath, individuals can shift their attention away from pain and cultivate a sense of calm.
3. Mindful Movement: Mindful movement practices, such as gentle yoga or tai chi, combine mindfulness with physical

activity. These practices encourage individuals to move with awareness, focusing on the sensations of movement and breath. This can help improve flexibility, reduce pain, and promote a sense of body connection.

4. Guided Meditation: Guided meditations can provide a structured approach to mindfulness practice. Listening to a guided meditation can help individuals focus on specific aspects of their pain experience, promoting acceptance, relaxation, and a sense of control over their pain.

5.   Mindful Self-Compassion: Mindful self-compassion practices involve extending kindness and understanding towards oneself, even in the face of chronic pain. This can help reduce self-criticism and promote self-acceptance, which can in turn improve overall well-being and pain management.

Incorporating mindfulness techniques into daily life can significantly improve chronic pain management. Here are some tips for integrating mindfulness into your routine:

1. Start with short sessions: Begin with brief mindfulness practices, such as a few minutes of mindful breathing, and gradually increase the duration as you feel more comfortable.

2.   Find a quiet and comfortable space: Choose a quiet, distraction-free environment where you can practise mindfulness without interruptions.

3. Be patient and consistent: Mindfulness requires practice and patience. Don't be discouraged if you find it challenging at first. Consistent practice is key to reaping the benefits.

4. Seek guidance from a qualified teacher: Consider working with a mindfulness teacher or attending mindfulness-based stress reduction (MBSR) classes to learn proper techniques and receive support.

5. Cmbine with other modalities: Integrate mindfulness into your existing chronic pain management plan, working with

your healthcare provider to determine the most effective approach for you.

Mindfulness offers a safe, non-invasive, and effective way to manage chronic pain, promoting physical and mental relief. By incorporating mindfulness techniques into your daily routine, you can enhance your overall well-being, reduce pain intensity, and improve your ability to cope with chronic pain.

How To Find A Yoga Class Or Mindfulness Teacher

Finding a suitable yoga class or mindfulness teacher for someone with chronic pain can make a significant difference in managing their condition and improving their overall well-being. Here's a step-by-step guide to finding the right fit:

1. Seek recommendations: Ask your healthcare provider, physical therapist, or support group members for recommendations of yoga instructors or mindfulness teachers with experience in working with individuals with chronic pain.
2. Check online resources: Search online directories, such as Yoga Alliance or the International Association of Yoga Therapists, to find instructors or teachers in your area who specialise in chronic pain management.
3. Consider their qualifications: Ensure the instructor or teacher has appropriate training and certifications in yoga or mindfulness, preferably with a focus on chronic pain management.
4. Read reviews and testimonials: Read online reviews and testimonials from previous students to get a sense of the instructor's or teacher's teaching style and effectiveness in managing chronic pain.
5. Contact the instructor or teacher: Contact the instructor

or teacher directly to discuss your specific needs and limitations related to chronic pain. Ask about their experience with chronic pain and how they modify poses or techniques to suit individual needs.

6.   Attend a trial class: If possible, attend a trial class or introductory session to experience the instructor's or teacher's teaching style and the overall atmosphere of the class. Observe how they interact with students and address their needs.

7. Ask about modifications: Inquire about the instructor's or teacher's approach to modifications and how they adapt poses or techniques to accommodate individuals with chronic pain.

8. Cmmunicate your needs: Clearly communicate your pain levels, limitations, and any specific concerns you have to the instructor or teacher before starting classes.

9. Trust your instincts: Choose an instructor or teacher who makes you feel comfortable, respected, and confident in their ability to support your chronic pain management journey.

Remember, finding the right yoga class or mindfulness teacher requires patience and exploration. Don't hesitate to try different instructors or teachers until you find one who aligns with your needs and preferences. Consistent practice with a qualified instructor or teacher can significantly improve your chronic pain management and enhance your overall well-being.

CHAPTER 5: OTHER ALTERNATIVE AND COMPLEMENTARY THERAPIES

"Pain is a part of life, but it does not have to control your life. You can choose to let pain consume you, or you can choose to rise above it." - Nicole Davis

Massage Therapy

Massage therapy is a form of complementary and alternative medicine (CAM) that involves applying pressure to muscles, tendons, and ligaments to promote relaxation, reduce pain, and improve circulation. It has been used for centuries to treat a wide range of conditions, including chronic pain.

Benefits of Massage Therapy for Chronic Pain

Massage therapy can offer several benefits for individuals with chronic pain, including:

1. Pain Reduction: Massage can help to reduce pain by

stimulating the release of endorphins, the body's natural painkillers. It can also improve muscle circulation and reduce muscle tension, which can further contribute to pain relief.

2. Improved Relaxation: Massage can promote relaxation by triggering the parasympathetic nervous system, which is responsible for the body's "rest-and-digest" response. This can help to reduce stress hormones, improve sleep quality, and alleviate anxiety associated with chronic pain.

3. Enhanced Circulation: Massage stimulates blood flow to the muscles, delivering oxygen and nutrients that support healing and muscle function. Improved circulation can also help to reduce muscle stiffness and discomfort.

4. Reduced Muscle Tension: Massage techniques can help to release muscle tension, alleviate muscle spasms, and improve flexibility. This can be particularly beneficial for individuals with chronic pain conditions like arthritis or fibromyalgia.

5. Enhanced Mood and Well-being: Massage can boost endorphins, which have mood-enhancing effects. Additionally, reducing stress and pain can contribute to an overall improvement in mood and well-being, leading to a better quality of life for individuals with chronic pain.

Types of Massage Therapy for Chronic Pain

Several massage therapy techniques are commonly used for chronic pain management, each with its unique approach and benefits:

1. Swedish Massage: A gentle, relaxing massage that uses long, smooth strokes to increase blood flow and release muscle tension. It is a good starting point for individuals new to massage therapy.

2. Deep Tissue Massage: A more intense massage that applies deeper pressure to reach muscles and connective tissues

beneath the surface. It is often used to treat chronic pain, muscle injuries, and trigger points.

3. Sports Massage: Specifically designed for athletes to help prepare for and recover from competition. It focuses on improving flexibility, range of motion, and muscle performance.

4. Trigger Point Massage: Targets trigger points, which are small, tight nodules in muscles that can cause pain. Trigger point massage aims to release these trigger points and reduce pain.

5. Thai Massage: Combines massage, stretching, and yoga techniques. Thai massage is known for its ability to improve flexibility, range of motion, and circulation.

Considerations for Massage Therapy

While massage therapy is generally safe for most people, it is essential to consider potential side effects and seek guidance before starting.

- Side Effects: Massage may cause temporary discomfort, such as soreness, bruising, or muscle aches. These side effects typically subside within a few days.
- Medical Conditions: Massage therapy may not be suitable for individuals with certain medical conditions, such as bleeding disorders, cancer, or infections. Consult your doctor before starting massage therapy if you have any underlying health concerns.
- Qualified Massage Therapist: Finding a qualified and experienced massage therapist is crucial. Ask for recommendations from your doctor or search for certified massage therapists in your area.

In conclusion, massage therapy can serve as a valuable complementary and alternative therapy for managing chronic pain. By promoting relaxation, reducing pain, and improving circulation, massage can contribute to an overall improvement in the quality of life for individuals living with chronic pain. However, it is essential to consult with your doctor and find a qualified massage therapist to ensure safe and effective treatment.

Acupuncture

Acupuncture is a form of traditional Chinese medicine (TCM) that involves inserting thin needles into specific points on the body to stimulate energy flow, also known as qi or vital energy. It has been used for centuries to treat a wide range of conditions, including chronic pain.

Benefits of Acupuncture for Chronic Pain

Acupuncture has been shown to be effective for managing chronic pain from various conditions, including:

- Lower back pain: Acupuncture can help reduce pain and improve function in individuals with lower back pain, both acute and chronic.
- Neck pain: Acupuncture can alleviate pain and improve neck mobility in individuals suffering from neck pain.
- Osteoarthritis: Acupuncture can help reduce pain and improve joint function in individuals with osteoarthritis, a degenerative joint disease.
- Fibromyalgia: Acupuncture can help reduce pain, fatigue, and sleep disturbances associated with fibromyalgia.
- Headaches: Acupuncture can help prevent and reduce the frequency and intensity of headaches, particularly migraines.

Mechanism of Action

The precise mechanism of acupuncture's pain-relieving effects is still being investigated, but several theories have been proposed:

- Stimulation of endorphin release: Acupuncture may

stimulate the release of endorphins, the body's natural painkillers, which can help reduce pain perception.

- Modulation of pain signals: Acupuncture may modulate neurotransmitter activity, influencing the transmission of pain signals in the spinal cord and brain.
- Anti-inflammatory effects: Acupuncture may have anti-inflammatory properties, reducing inflammation that can contribute to chronic pain.
- Improvement of blood flow: Acupuncture may improve blood circulation to affected areas, promoting healing and reducing pain.
- Activation of the parasympathetic nervous system: Acupuncture may activate the parasympathetic nervous system, which is responsible for the body's "rest-and-digest" response, promoting relaxation and reducing stress hormones.

Types of Acupuncture

There are various styles and techniques of acupuncture, each with its unique approach and emphasis:

- Traditional Chinese acupuncture: The most common form, based on TCM principles and using specific points on the body to balance qi flow.
- Electroacupuncture: Combines traditional acupuncture with electrical stimulation of acupuncture needles to enhance the therapeutic effects.
- Auricular acupuncture: Focuses on points on the ear, particularly for pain management and addiction treatment.
- Five-element acupuncture: Emphasises the balance of five elements (wood, fire, earth, metal, and water) to address pain and other health concerns.
- Shonishin: A Japanese acupuncture technique using very fine needles and shallow insertion, often used for pain management in children.

Safety Considerations

Acupuncture is generally considered safe when administered by a qualified acupuncturist. However, potential side effects may include:

- Temporary discomfort: Some individuals may experience mild discomfort or soreness at the acupuncture points.
- Minor bleeding: Minor bleeding at the insertion sites is possible but usually subsides quickly.
- Bruising: Bruising at the acupuncture points may occur occasionally.
- Rare side effects: In rare cases, more serious side effects like organ puncture or infection may occur, but these are extremely uncommon when proper techniques and sterile needles are used.

Finding a Qualified Acupuncturist

It is crucial to find a qualified and experienced acupuncturist to ensure safe and effective treatment. Seek recommendations from your doctor or search for certified acupuncturists in your area. Check their credentials, experience, and specialisation in pain management.

In conclusion, acupuncture offers a promising complementary and alternative therapy for managing chronic pain. By stimulating the body's natural healing mechanisms and addressing pain at its root cause, acupuncture can provide relief and improve overall well-being for individuals living with chronic pain. However, it is essential to consult with your doctor and find a qualified acupuncturist to ensure a safe and effective treatment plan.

Chiropractic Care

Chiropractic care is a form of complementary and alternative medicine (CAM) that involves manipulating the spine to improve alignment, relieve pain, and enhance overall health. It is based on the principle that misalignment of the spine can interfere with the nervous system and contribute to various health problems, including chronic pain.

Benefits of Chiropractic Care for Chronic Pain

Chiropractic care has been shown to be effective for managing chronic pain from various conditions, including:

- Low back pain: Chiropractic adjustments can help reduce pain and improve function in individuals with lower back pain, both acute and chronic.
- Neck pain: Chiropractic manipulations can alleviate pain and improve neck mobility in individuals suffering from neck pain.
- Headaches: Chiropractic care may help prevent and reduce the frequency and intensity of headaches, particularly migraines.
- Arthritis: Chiropractic adjustments may help reduce pain and improve joint function in individuals with arthritis, particularly osteoarthritis.
- Other musculoskeletal conditions: Chiropractic care may be beneficial for other musculoskeletal conditions, such as fibromyalgia, carpal tunnel syndrome, and sciatica.

Mechanism of Action

The precise mechanism of chiropractic care's pain-relieving effects is still being investigated, but several theories have been proposed:

- Spinal manipulation and alignment: Chiropractic adjustments aim to restore proper alignment of the spine, which may alleviate pressure on nerve roots and reduce pain signals.

- Stimulation of endorphin release: Chiropractic manipulations may stimulate the release of endorphins, the body's natural painkillers, which can help reduce pain perception.
- Improved muscle function and flexibility: Chiropractic adjustments may improve muscle function and flexibility, reducing muscle spasms and enhancing range of motion, which can contribute to pain relief.
- Reduced inflammation: Chiropractic manipulations may have anti-inflammatory properties, reducing inflammation that can contribute to chronic pain.
- Activation of the parasympathetic nervous system: Chiropractic care may activate the parasympathetic nervous system, which is responsible for the body's "rest-and-digest" response, promoting relaxation and reducing stress hormones.

Types of Chiropractic Techniques

There are various techniques and approaches within chiropractic care, each with its unique emphasis and application:

- Diversified technique: The most common chiropractic approach, using a combination of manual adjustments, stretching, and soft tissue manipulation.
- Spinal manipulative therapy: A broad term encompassing various techniques that involve manipulation of the spine to improve alignment and function.
- Gonstead technique: A specific chiropractic technique that emphasises precise and controlled adjustments based on X-ray analysis.
- Activator technique: A low-force chiropractic technique that uses a spring-loaded instrument to deliver precise adjustments.
- Sacro-occipital technique (SOT): A chiropractic technique that focuses on balancing the pelvis and the sacrum, the

triangular bone at the base of the spine.

Safety Considerations

Chiropractic care is generally considered safe when administered by a qualified chiropractor. However, potential side effects may include:

- Temporary discomfort: Some individuals may experience mild discomfort or soreness after chiropractic adjustments.
- Minor headaches: Minor headaches may occur occasionally following adjustments.
- Temporary muscle stiffness: Muscle stiffness may be experienced temporarily after adjustments.
- Rare side effects: In rare cases, more serious side effects like pinched nerves or herniated discs may occur, but these are extremely uncommon when proper techniques are used.

Finding a Qualified Chiropractor

It is crucial to find a qualified and experienced chiropractor to ensure safe and effective treatment. Seek recommendations from your doctor or search for certified chiropractors in your area. Check their credentials, experience, and specialisation in pain management.

In conclusion, chiropractic care can be a valuable complementary and alternative therapy for managing chronic pain. By addressing misalignment of the spine and promoting overall musculoskeletal health, chiropractic care can provide pain relief, improve function, and enhance the quality of life for individuals living with chronic pain. However, it is essential to consult with your doctor and find a qualified chiropractor to ensure a safe and effective treatment plan.

Biofeedback

Biofeedback is a form of complementary and alternative medicine (CAM) that involves gaining control over certain involuntary bodily functions, such as heart rate, muscle tension, and blood pressure. It is based on the principle that by monitoring these physiological processes and providing feedback, individuals can learn to regulate them, leading to improved health outcomes.

Benefits of Biofeedback for Chronic Pain

Biofeedback has been shown to be effective for managing chronic pain from various conditions, including:

- Musculoskeletal pain: Biofeedback can help reduce muscle tension, improve flexibility, and enhance range of motion, which can contribute to pain relief in conditions like lower back pain, neck pain, and fibromyalgia.
- Headaches: Biofeedback may help prevent and reduce the frequency and intensity of headaches, particularly migraines.
- Neuropathic pain: Biofeedback can be beneficial for neuropathic pain, which arises from damage or dysfunction of the nervous system, such as pain caused by diabetic neuropathy or shingles.
- Visceral pain: Biofeedback may help manage visceral pain, which originates from internal organs, such as abdominal pain or pelvic pain.
- Stress-related pain: Biofeedback can help reduce stress and anxiety, which can exacerbate chronic pain symptoms.

Mechanism of Action

Biofeedback's pain-relieving effects are attributed to several mechanisms:

- Increased awareness and self-control: Biofeedback provides individuals with real-time feedback about their bodily functions, allowing them to become more aware of their pain triggers and develop strategies to regulate them.

- Relaxation and stress reduction: Biofeedback techniques, such as deep breathing exercises and progressive muscle relaxation, can promote relaxation and reduce stress hormones, which can contribute to pain reduction.
- Neuromodulation: Biofeedback may influence the activity of the nervous system, modulating pain signals and reducing pain perception.
- Improved self-efficacy and empowerment: Biofeedback can enhance self-efficacy, the belief in one's ability to control their pain, which can empower individuals to manage their condition more effectively.

Types of Biofeedback

Biofeedback encompasses various techniques that target different physiological processes:

- Electromyography (EMG) biofeedback: Monitors muscle tension, helping individuals learn to relax muscles and reduce muscle spasms.
- Electroencephalography (EEG) biofeedback: Measures brainwave activity, helping individuals learn to regulate their mental state and reduce stress.
- Heart rate variability (HRV) biofeedback: Monitors heart rate variability, providing feedback on the balance between the sympathetic and parasympathetic nervous systems.
- Skin conductance biofeedback: Measures skin conductance, an indicator of sweat gland activity, which can reflect emotional arousal and stress levels.
- Temperature biofeedback: Monitors skin temperature, providing feedback on blood flow and relaxation levels.

Safety Considerations

Biofeedback is generally considered safe when administered by a qualified biofeedback therapist. However, potential side effects may include:

- Temporary discomfort: Some individuals may experience mild discomfort or dizziness during biofeedback sessions.
- Frustration and discouragement: Biofeedback may require patience and practice, and some individuals may experience frustration or discouragement if they don't see immediate results.
- Rare side effects: In rare cases, adverse reactions may occur, such as anxiety or panic attacks, but these are extremely uncommon when proper techniques are used.

Finding a Qualified Biofeedback Therapist

It is crucial to find a qualified and experienced biofeedback therapist to ensure safe and effective treatment. Seek recommendations from your doctor or search for certified biofeedback therapists in your area. Check their credentials, experience, and specialisation in pain management.

In conclusion, biofeedback offers a promising complementary and alternative therapy for managing chronic pain. By providing individuals with control over their bodily functions and promoting relaxation, biofeedback can help reduce pain symptoms, improve function, and enhance overall well-being. However, it is essential to consult with your doctor and find a qualified biofeedback therapist to ensure a safe and effective treatment plan.

Relaxation Techniques

Relaxation techniques are a form of complementary and alternative medicine (CAM) that involve various methods to promote relaxation, reduce stress, and manage pain. These techniques aim to create a sense of calm and tranquillity, which can help alleviate pain symptoms and improve overall well-being.

Benefits of Relaxation Techniques for Chronic Pain

Relaxation techniques have shown significant benefits in managing chronic pain from various conditions, including:

- Musculoskeletal pain: Relaxation techniques can help reduce muscle tension, improve flexibility, and enhance range of motion, contributing to pain relief in conditions like lower back pain, neck pain, and fibromyalgia.
- Headaches: Relaxation techniques may help prevent and reduce the frequency and intensity of headaches, particularly migraines.
- Neuropathic pain: Relaxation techniques can be beneficial for neuropathic pain, which arises from damage or dysfunction of the nervous system, such as pain caused by diabetic neuropathy or shingles.
- Visceral pain: Relaxation techniques may help manage visceral pain, which originates from internal organs, such as abdominal pain or pelvic pain.
- Stress-related pain: Relaxation techniques can help reduce stress and anxiety, which can exacerbate chronic pain symptoms.

Mechanism of Action

Relaxation techniques work by influencing the nervous system and physiological processes in several ways:

- Activation of the parasympathetic nervous system: Relaxation techniques promote the parasympathetic nervous system's "rest-and-digest" response, which reduces stress hormones and promotes relaxation.
- Reduction of muscle tension: Relaxation techniques, such as deep breathing and progressive muscle relaxation, can help reduce muscle tension and spasms, contributing to pain relief.

- Improved blood flow: Relaxation techniques can promote better blood flow to affected areas, delivering oxygen and nutrients to aid healing and reduce pain.
- Pain gate theory: Relaxation techniques may influence the pain gate, a mechanism in the spinal cord that controls pain signals travelling to the brain. Relaxation can help open the pain gate, reducing pain perception.
- Mind-body connection: Relaxation techniques promote a sense of mind-body connection, allowing individuals to become more aware of their thoughts, feelings, and bodily sensations, which can help them better manage their pain.

Types of Relaxation Techniques

Numerous relaxation techniques can be used to manage chronic pain, each with its unique approach and benefits:

- Deep breathing exercises: Deep, slow breathing can activate the parasympathetic nervous system and reduce stress hormones, promoting relaxation and pain relief.
- Progressive muscle relaxation: This technique involves tensing and relaxing different muscle groups throughout the body, helping to release muscle tension and promote relaxation.
- Guided imagery: This involves using visualisation techniques to imagine relaxing environments or scenarios, promoting a sense of calm and reducing stress.
- Meditation: Meditation focuses on calming the mind and reducing distracting thoughts, promoting relaxation and self-awareness.
- Mindfulness: As described above, mindfulness involves paying attention to the present moment without judgement, fostering acceptance and reducing stress that can exacerbate pain.
- Yoga: As described above, yoga combines physical postures, breathing exercises, and meditation, promoting flexibility,

relaxation, and stress reduction.

- Tai chi: Tai chi involves slow, gentle movements and deep breathing, promoting relaxation, balance, and stress reduction.

Safety Considerations

Relaxation techniques are generally safe when practised appropriately. However, it is important to consider potential side effects and consult with a healthcare professional before starting any new relaxation technique, especially if you have any underlying health conditions.

- Temporary discomfort: Some individuals may experience mild discomfort or dizziness during relaxation techniques, such as deep breathing or meditation.
- Emotional processing: Relaxation techniques can sometimes trigger emotional responses, such as sadness or anger, as individuals become more aware of their emotions. It is essential to allow these emotions to arise and process them in a healthy way.
- Over-relaxation: In rare cases, individuals may experience excessive relaxation or drowsiness, particularly with techniques like deep breathing or meditation. It is important to adjust the practice to a comfortable level and avoid situations where over-relaxation could be dangerous.

Finding a Qualified Instructor or Therapist

As always, if you are considering using relaxation techniques for chronic pain management, it is advisable to seek guidance from a qualified instructor or therapist. Look for individuals with experience in teaching relaxation techniques for pain management and ensure they have appropriate training and credentials.

In conclusion, relaxation techniques offer a safe, effective, and non-invasive approach to managing chronic pain. By promoting relaxation, reducing stress, and enhancing mind-body connection, these techniques can help alleviate pain symptoms, improve function, and enhance overall well-being. However, it is essential to consult with your healthcare provider and find a qualified instructor or therapist to ensure safe and effective practice.

CHAPTER 6: SELF-MANAGEMENT STRATEGIES FOR CHRONIC PAIN

"Pain is not the end; it is a new beginning. It is the opportunity to learn and grow, to become stronger and more resilient." - Jenni Schaefer

Setting Realistic Goals

Setting realistic goals is an essential self-management strategy for individuals living with chronic pain. Chronic pain can be a debilitating condition that significantly impacts daily life, making it crucial to develop effective coping mechanisms and strategies to manage pain and maintain a sense of well-being.

Importance of Setting Realistic Goals

Goal setting plays a vital role in chronic pain management for several reasons:

1. Provides Direction and Motivation: Setting goals provides a

clear direction and sense of purpose, helping individuals stay motivated and focused on their pain management journey.

2. Promotes Self-Empowerment: Setting achievable goals fosters a sense of self-efficacy and empowerment, encouraging individuals to take ownership of their pain management and believe in their ability to make progress.

3. Measures Progress and Success: Setting goals allows individuals to track their progress, celebrate achievements, and make adjustments as needed, providing a sense of accomplishment and reinforcing positive behaviour change.

Steps to Setting Realistic Goals

1. Identify Areas of Improvement: Reflect on the areas of life most impacted by chronic pain and identify specific aspects you would like to improve.

2. Define Clear and Measurable Goals: Formulate specific, measurable, achievable, relevant, and time-bound (SMART) goals. For example, instead of aiming to "reduce pain," set a goal like "reduce pain intensity by 20% in the next three months."

3. Break Down Goals into Smaller Steps: Divide large goals into smaller, more manageable steps to make them less overwhelming and increase the likelihood of success.

4. Consider Your Limitations: Be realistic about your physical and emotional limitations, and set goals that are challenging but achievable within your current abilities.

5. Set Realistic Timelines: Establish realistic timelines for each goal, considering the complexity and effort required. Avoid setting unrealistic deadlines that may lead to discouragement.

Examples of Realistic Goals for Chronic Pain Management

1. Physical Activity: Set goals for regular physical activity, gradually increasing the duration and intensity as tolerated.

2. Stress Management: Incorporate stress-reducing techniques

like yoga, meditation, or deep breathing into your routine.

3.   Sleep Hygiene: Establish a consistent sleep schedule, create a relaxing bedtime routine, and avoid caffeine and alcohol before bed.
4.   Dietary Habits: Make gradual changes to your diet, incorporating more fruits, vegetables, and whole grains while limiting processed foods and sugary drinks.
5.   Pain Coping Strategies: Identify and practise effective pain coping strategies, such as relaxation techniques, mindfulness, or cognitive-behavioural therapy (CBT).

Tips for Staying Motivated

1.   Track Your Progress: Keep a journal or progress chart to monitor your achievements, no matter how small. Celebrating milestones can boost motivation.
2.   Seek Support: Surround yourself with supportive individuals, join support groups, or seek professional guidance to stay motivated and accountable.
3.   Reward Yourself: Acknowledge and reward yourself for reaching goals, reinforcing positive behaviour and maintaining motivation.
4.   Adjust Goals as Needed: Life circumstances change, so be flexible and adjust your goals as needed to ensure they remain realistic and achievable.
5.   Focus on the Journey: Chronic pain management is an ongoing process, so focus on making consistent progress rather than striving for instant perfection.

Remember, setting realistic goals is a powerful tool for self-management and can significantly improve your quality of life with chronic pain. By establishing clear goals, breaking them down into manageable steps, and tracking your progress, you can take control of your pain management journey and achieve meaningful improvements in your daily life.

Pacing Your Activities

Pacing your activities is a crucial self-management strategy for individuals living with chronic pain. Chronic pain can significantly impact energy levels and stamina, making it essential to manage activities wisely to avoid overexertion and worsening pain symptoms.

Importance of Pacing Activities

Pacing your activities offers several benefits for chronic pain management:

1. Reduces Pain Exacerbations: By avoiding overexertion, pacing helps prevent pain flare-ups and reduces the intensity and duration of pain episodes.
2. Enhances Energy Levels: Pacing allows you to distribute your energy throughout the day, preventing fatigue and enabling you to engage in activities you enjoy without feeling drained.
3. Promotes Consistency: Pacing encourages consistency in your daily routine, helping you maintain a sense of normalcy and avoid feeling overwhelmed by pain.
4. Improves Overall Well-being: By managing activity levels effectively, pacing can contribute to improved physical and emotional well-being, reducing stress and anxiety associated with chronic pain.

Principles of Pacing Activities

1. Identify Your Limits: Recognize your physical and emotional limitations and set realistic expectations for what you can accomplish without experiencing pain flare-ups.
2. Start Gradually: Begin with short, low-impact activities and gradually increase the duration and intensity as tolerated. Avoid pushing yourself beyond your limits.

3. Prioritise Activities: Identify the most important activities that you want to be able to do consistently and allocate your energy accordingly.
4. Balance Activity with Rest: Schedule regular rest periods throughout the day to allow your body to recover and prevent fatigue.
5. Listen to Your Body: Pay attention to your body's signals. If you experience pain or fatigue, stop the activity and rest.
6. Break Down Activities: Divide large tasks into smaller, more manageable steps to avoid feeling overwhelmed and conserve energy.
7. Incorporate Flexibility: Be flexible and willing to adjust your plans based on your pain levels and energy levels on a given day.
8. Seek Support: Encourage friends, family, or a healthcare professional to help you monitor your activity levels and provide assistance when needed.

Tips for Pacing Activities

1. Use a Timer: Set a timer to manage the duration of activities and avoid overexertion.
2. Alternate Activities: Alternate between high-energy activities and low-energy activities to balance your energy expenditure.
3. Incorporate Pacing into Daily Routine: Make pacing a regular part of your daily routine, scheduling rest periods and managing activity levels consistently.
4. Track Your Progress: Monitor your progress and make adjustments to your pacing strategies as needed.
5. Seek Professional Guidance: Consult a physical therapist or occupational therapist to develop a personalised pacing plan tailored to your specific needs and limitations.

Remember, pacing your activities is an ongoing process that requires self-awareness, flexibility, and a willingness to adjust your approach as needed. By effectively managing your activity levels, you can significantly reduce pain flare-ups, improve your energy levels, and enhance your overall well-being, enabling you to live a more fulfilling life despite chronic pain.

Identifying And Avoiding Pain Triggers

Identifying and avoiding pain triggers is a crucial self-management strategy for individuals living with chronic pain. Chronic pain can be triggered by various factors, including physical activities, emotional stress, environmental conditions, and lifestyle habits. By recognizing and avoiding these triggers, individuals can significantly reduce pain flare-ups and improve their overall well-being.

Importance of Identifying and Avoiding Pain Triggers

Identifying and avoiding pain triggers offers several benefits for chronic pain management:

1.   Reduces Pain Flare-ups: By avoiding known triggers, individuals can minimise the frequency and intensity of pain flare-ups.
2. Improves Pain Control: Understanding and avoiding triggers enhances pain control, allowing individuals to manage their condition more effectively.
3. Promotes Self-Awareness: Identifying triggers fosters self-awareness, empowering individuals to take proactive steps to manage their pain.
4. Enhances Overall Well-being: By reducing pain flare-ups and improving pain control, avoiding triggers can contribute to improved physical, emotional, and social well-being.

Steps to Identify Pain Triggers

1. Keep a Pain Journal: Record the occurrence of pain episodes,

including the time, intensity, and any activities, emotions, or environmental factors that may have preceded the pain.

2. Recognise Patterns: Identify patterns in your pain journal, noting any recurring triggers or associations between pain and specific activities, emotions, or environments.
3. Seek Professional Guidance: Consult a healthcare professional to discuss potential triggers and receive personalised advice on identifying and avoiding them.

Common Pain Triggers

1. Physical Activities: Certain physical activities, such as lifting heavy objects, prolonged sitting or standing, or engaging in repetitive movements, may trigger pain.
2. Emotional Stress: Stress, anxiety, and negative emotions can exacerbate pain symptoms.
3. Environmental Conditions: Weather changes, exposure to cold or humidity, or loud noises may trigger pain.
4. Lifestyle Habits: Poor sleep habits, smoking, alcohol consumption, and unhealthy dietary choices can contribute to pain.
5. Medical Conditions: Underlying medical conditions, such as arthritis, fibromyalgia, or migraines, may have specific triggers.

Strategies for Avoiding Pain Triggers

1. Modify Activities: Alter or avoid activities that consistently trigger pain flare-ups.
2. Manage Stress: Implement stress management techniques, such as relaxation exercises, yoga, or meditation, to reduce stress levels and minimise pain triggers.
3. Control Environmental Factors: Adapt your environment to minimise known triggers, such as adjusting temperature, using noise-cancelling headphones, or avoiding exposure to irritants.
4. Maintain Healthy Habits: Adopt healthy lifestyle habits,

including regular exercise, a balanced diet, and adequate sleep, to promote overall well-being and reduce pain susceptibility, see above where these topics are dealt with in more detail.

5. Seek Medical Intervention: Address underlying medical conditions with appropriate medical care to reduce the likelihood of pain triggers.

Remember, identifying and avoiding pain triggers is an individualised process that requires ongoing self-awareness and adaptation. By working with a healthcare professional, you can develop a personalised plan to identify your triggers and implement strategies to manage them effectively, improving your pain control and overall quality of life.

Getting Enough Sleep

Getting enough sleep is a crucial self-management strategy for individuals living with chronic pain. Sleep disturbances are a common symptom of chronic pain, and inadequate sleep can worsen pain symptoms, reduce energy levels, and impair overall well-being.

Importance of Adequate Sleep for Chronic Pain Management

1. Reduced Pain Perception: Adequate sleep promotes the release of pain-relieving hormones and reduces the production of stress hormones, which can contribute to pain perception.
2. Improved Mood and Energy Levels: Sufficient sleep enhances mood, reduces irritability, and improves energy levels, allowing individuals to better manage pain and engage in daily activities.
3. Enhanced Cognitive Function: Adequate sleep improves cognitive function, memory, and focus, which can help

individuals cope with pain more effectively.

4. Promotes Healing: Sleep plays a vital role in healing and repair processes, which can aid in managing pain and promoting overall health.

Recommended Sleep Duration for Adults

Most adults need around 7-8 hours of sleep per night to function optimally. However, individual sleep needs may vary, and individuals with chronic pain may require more sleep to manage their condition effectively.

Tips for Improving Sleep Quality for Chronic Pain

1. Establish a Regular Sleep Schedule: Set a consistent bedtime and wake-up time, even on weekends, to regulate your body's natural sleep-wake cycle.
2. Create a Relaxing Bedtime Routine: An hour or two before bed, engage in calming activities like reading, taking a warm bath, or listening to soothing music.
3. Optimise Your Sleep Environment: Ensure your bedroom is dark, quiet, and cool to promote restful sleep.
4. Avoid Caffeine and Alcohol: Avoid caffeine and alcohol close to bedtime, as they can interfere with sleep quality.
5. Regular Exercise: Engage in regular physical activity, following safety considerations laid out above, but try to avoid any strenuous exercise too close to bedtime.
6. Manage Stress: Implement stress management techniques like relaxation exercises, yoga, or meditation to reduce stress levels that can disrupt sleep, see above for more detail.
7. Seek Professional Help: If sleep disturbances persist despite lifestyle changes, consult a healthcare professional to rule out underlying medical conditions or sleep disorders.

Remember, getting enough sleep is an essential component of overall health, particularly for individuals living with chronic pain. By establishing healthy sleep habits and addressing any underlying sleep issues, you can improve sleep quality, reduce some pain symptoms, and enhance your overall well-being.

Managing Stress

Stress is a common symptom of chronic pain and can exacerbate pain symptoms, reduce energy levels, and impair overall well-being. Managing stress effectively is a crucial self-management strategy for individuals living with chronic pain.

Importance of Stress Management for Chronic Pain

1. Reduced Pain Perception: Stress can heighten pain perception and make pain symptoms more intense. Managing stress can help reduce pain intensity and improve pain control.
2. Improved Mood and Energy Levels: Chronic pain and stress can lead to fatigue and irritability. Effective stress management can enhance mood, increase energy levels, and improve overall well-being.
3. Enhanced Coping Mechanisms: Stress management techniques can equip individuals with coping mechanisms to handle pain and other challenges associated with chronic pain more effectively.
4. Reduced Anxiety and Depression: Chronic pain can increase the risk of anxiety and depression. Managing stress can help reduce these co-occurring conditions and promote emotional well-being.

Effective Stress Management Techniques

1. Relaxation Techniques: Engage in relaxation techniques such as deep breathing exercises, progressive muscle relaxation, or meditation to promote relaxation and reduce stress hormones.
2. Mindfulness: As described in more detail above, practise mindfulness to cultivate present-moment awareness and

reduce rumination on negative thoughts, which can contribute to stress and anxiety.

3. Regular Exercise: Engage in regular physical activity, subject to the safety considerations mentioned above, as exercise releases endorphins, which have mood-boosting and stress-reducing effects.

4. Social Support: Maintain strong social connections and seek support from friends, family, or support groups to reduce feelings of isolation and stress.

5. Cognitive Behavioral Therapy (CBT): Consider CBT, a type of therapy that helps identify and modify negative thought patterns that contribute to stress and anxiety.

6. Seek Professional Help: Consult a healthcare professional or therapist if stress management techniques alone are not effective in managing stress levels.

Remember, stress management is an ongoing process that requires consistent effort and self-awareness. By implementing effective stress management strategies, you can reduce the impact of stress on your chronic pain, improve your overall well-being, and enhance your quality of life.

Maintaining A Positive Outlook

Maintaining a positive outlook is a crucial self-management strategy for individuals living with chronic pain. While chronic pain can be challenging and disruptive, cultivating a positive mindset can significantly impact your ability to cope with pain, manage stress, and maintain overall well-being.

Benefits of a Positive Outlook for Chronic Pain Management

1. Enhanced Pain Coping: A positive outlook can improve your coping mechanisms and resilience in dealing with chronic pain, reducing the perceived intensity of pain symptoms.

2.   Improved Mood and Emotional Well-being: A positive mindset can elevate your mood, reduce anxiety and depression, and promote a sense of optimism, which can all contribute to better pain management.

3.   Increased Motivation and Adherence to Treatment: A positive outlook can enhance motivation to engage in self-management strategies, such as exercise, relaxation techniques, and healthy lifestyle choices.

4. Enhanced Quality of Life: A positive mindset can improve your overall quality of life, despite the challenges of chronic pain, allowing you to focus on enjoyable activities and maintain a sense of purpose.

Strategies for Cultivating a Positive Outlook

1.   Focus on Gratitude: Practise gratitude, where possible, by acknowledging and appreciating the positive aspects of your life, even small things like a good night's sleep or a supportive friend.

2. Challenge Negative Thoughts: Try to recognise and challenge negative thoughts that may contribute to stress and anxiety. Try to replace them with more realistic and positive self-talk.

3. Set Realistic and Achievable Goals: As detailed above, setting achievable goals, even small ones, can provide a sense of accomplishment and boost motivation, contributing to a more positive outlook.

4.   Engage in Activities You Enjoy: Schedule time for activities that bring you joy and fulfilment, whether it's hobbies, spending time with loved ones, or pursuing creative endeavours.

5.   Seek Support: Surround yourself with supportive individuals who uplift and encourage you. Join support groups or connect with others who understand the challenges of chronic pain.

6.   Seek Professional Help: Consider seeking professional guidance from a therapist or counsellor if you struggle with

maintaining a positive outlook on your own.

Remember, cultivating a positive outlook is an ongoing process that requires consistent effort and self-awareness. By incorporating positive mindset practices into your daily life, you can significantly enhance your ability to cope with chronic pain, improve your overall well-being, and live a more fulfilling life.

CHAPTER 7: RESOURCES FOR FURTHER INFORMATION

"Pain is not a weakness; it is a part of what makes us human. It is through our pain that we learn empathy, compassion, and strength."
- Maya Angelou

Organisations That Provide Support For People With Chronic Pain

Organisations that provide support for people with chronic pain include:

- The American Chronic Pain Association (ACPA) is a national organisation that provides education, support, and advocacy for people living with chronic pain. The ACPA provides a wealth of information on chronic pain, including articles, videos, and a pain diary app. There is also a website with information on chronic pain conditions, treatment options, and self-management strategies. They also have a toll-free helpline that provides support and guidance to people with chronic pain and their families.

https://www.acpanow.com/

- The Chronic Pain Management Initiative (CPMI) is a joint initiative of the Harvard Medical School and the Massachusetts General Hospital that aims to improve the lives of people with chronic pain. The CPMI offers a variety of resources, including a website with information on chronic pain conditions, treatment options, and self-management strategies. They also have a blog that features articles on a variety of topics related to chronic pain, a podcast and a pain management toolkit.

  https://els.cpm.org/

- The European Pain Federation (EFIC) is a non-profit organisation that represents the interests of people with chronic pain in Europe. EFIC provides a variety of resources, including a website with information in multiple languages on specific chronic pain conditions, treatment options, and self-management strategies. They also have a blog that features articles on a variety of topics related to chronic pain. https://europeanpainfederation.eu/

- The International Association for the Study of Pain (IASP) is a professional organisation that promotes research, education, and clinical practice in the field of pain. The IASP offers a variety of resources, including a website with information on chronic pain conditions, treatment options, and self-management strategies for both patients and healthcare professionals. They also have a journal that publishes research on pain.

https://www.iasp-pain.org/

- The Pain Action Alliance of Advocates (PAIN Action) is a

national advocacy organisation that works to improve the lives of people with chronic pain. PAIN Action provides a variety of resources, including a website with information on chronic pain conditions, management and treatment options, advocacy strategies and pain related legislation. They also have a toll-free helpline that provides support and guidance to people with chronic pain and their families. https://action-on-pain.co.uk/

In addition to these national organisations, there are many local and regional organisations that provide support for people with chronic pain. You can find a list of local organisations in your area by searching online or contacting your local pain clinic or hospital.

Here are some additional resources that may be helpful:

- The National Institute of Neurological Disorders and Stroke (NINDS) is a part of the National Institutes of Health (NIH) and provides information on a variety of neurological disorders, including chronic pain. The NINDS website has a section on chronic pain that includes information on symptoms, diagnosis, treatment, and research.

  https://www.ninds.nih.gov/

- The National Institute of Arthritis and Musculoskeletal and Skin Diseases (NIAMS) is a part of the NIH and provides information on a variety of musculoskeletal diseases, including chronic pain. The NIAMS website has a section on chronic pain that includes information on symptoms, causes, diagnosis, treatment, and research.

  https://www.niams.nih.gov/

- The National Center for Complementary and Integrative Health (NCCIH) is a part of the NIH and provides information on complementary and integrative health (CAM) therapies, including those that may be helpful for chronic pain. The

NCCIH website has a section on chronic pain that includes information on CAM therapies, self-management strategies, and research.

https://www.nccih.nih.gov/

- **Books and websites on chronic pain**

Books

The Real Meal Revolution: The Noakes Foundation Guide to Low-Carb, High-Fat Eating by Tim Noakes

This book provides a way of life that minimises the effects of inflammatory foods on the body.

Pain Free: A Revolutionary Approach to Chronic Pain by Dr. Deepak Ravindran

This book provides a comprehensive overview of chronic pain and offers practical advice on how to manage it using a variety of techniques, including mindfulness, relaxation, and cognitive-behavioural therapy.

Overcoming Chronic Pain: A Comprehensive Guide to Living Well with Pain by Dr. Frances Cole

This book offers a practical guide to managing chronic pain, covering topics such as understanding pain, setting goals, and managing stress.

Mind Over Pain: Rewiring the Brain to Break Free from Chronic Pain by Dr. John Sarno

This book discusses the role of the mind in chronic pain and offers techniques for rewiring the brain to reduce pain symptoms.

The Pain Zone: A Beginner's Guide to Chronic Pain by Dr. Paul St. Amand

This book provides a basic overview of chronic pain and its treatment, written in an easy-to-understand style.

The Miracle of Self-Healing: The Essential Guide to Healing Yourself from Chronic Pain and Illness by Dr. David Servan-Schreiber

This book offers a holistic approach to healing chronic pain, incorporating physical, mental, and emotional aspects of well-being.

In addition to these general resources, there are many websites that focus on specific pain conditions. For example, if you have fibromyalgia, you can find information on fibromyalgia-specific websites and support groups.

- **Clinical trials for chronic pain treatments**

Clinical trials are a crucial part of the medical research process, allowing scientists to evaluate the safety and efficacy of new treatments for various conditions, including chronic pain. Chronic pain affects millions of people worldwide, and ongoing research aims to develop more effective and tolerable treatment options.

Types of Clinical Trials for Chronic Pain

Clinical trials for chronic pain treatments can be categorised into different phases based on their objectives and the stage of development of the treatment being investigated:

- Phase 1 trials: These initial trials assess the safety and tolerability of a new treatment in a small group of healthy volunteers or patients with the target condition.
- Phase 2 trials: These trials evaluate the effectiveness of a treatment in a larger group of patients with the target condition, focusing on its ability to improve pain symptoms and overall well-being.
- Phase 3 trials: These large-scale trials compare the safety and efficacy of a new treatment against the standard of care or a placebo in a large group of patients.

- Phase 4 trials: These post-approval studies monitor the long-term safety and effectiveness of an approved treatment in a real-world setting.

Examples of Clinical Trials for Chronic Pain Treatments

Numerous clinical trials are currently underway to investigate various treatment approaches for chronic pain. Some examples include:

- New Medications: Researchers are developing new drugs targeting specific pain pathways or mechanisms, such as neuropathic pain medications, non-opioid analgesics, and anti-inflammatory agents.
- Neuromodulation Therapies: Clinical trials are evaluating the efficacy of neuromodulation techniques, such as deep brain stimulation, spinal cord stimulation, and transcranial magnetic stimulation, for managing chronic pain.
- Mind-Body Therapies: Studies are investigating the effectiveness of mind-body approaches, such as mindfulness-based stress reduction, cognitive-behavioural therapy, and yoga, in alleviating chronic pain symptoms.
- Complementary and Integrative Health (CAM) Therapies: Clinical trials are assessing the safety and efficacy of CAM therapies, such as acupuncture, massage therapy, and herbal remedies, for chronic pain management.

Finding and Participating in Clinical Trials

If you are interested in participating in a clinical trial for chronic pain treatment, several resources can help you find suitable opportunities:

- www.ClinicalTrials.gov: This website maintained by the National Institutes of Health (NIH) provides a comprehensive database of clinical trials worldwide.
- Patient Advocate Networks: Organisations like the ACPA and

PAIN Action, see details above, maintain lists of ongoing clinical trials and provide support to potential participants.

- Healthcare Provider Guidance: Consult your doctor or pain specialist to discuss potential clinical trials that align with your specific condition and treatment goals.

Considerations for Participating in Clinical Trials

Before participating in a clinical trial, it is essential to carefully consider the potential benefits and risks:

- Potential Benefits: The opportunity to receive an effective treatment before it becomes widely available, contribute to scientific research, and gain access to expert medical care.
- Potential Risks: The possibility of side effects or adverse reactions to the treatment, the uncertainty of treatment effectiveness, and the time commitment required for participation.

In conclusion, clinical trials play a vital role in advancing chronic pain treatments, offering hope for improved pain management and enhanced quality of life for individuals living with chronic pain. By participating in these trials, individuals can contribute to scientific progress and potentially gain access to new and effective treatment options.

ABOUT THE AUTHOR

Susan Robbie

Susan is a proud wife, mum, lawyer and sustainability consultant living in Somerset, in the United Kingdom. She is passionate about wildlife and social mobility and keen to make a difference in the world, which she finds beautiful and devastating in equal measure.

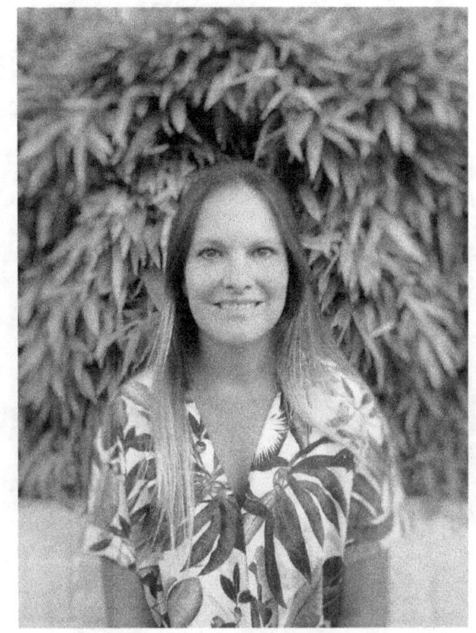